Created by <u>BabyDreamers.net</u>

Free Book Offer:

Get How to be a Super Mom For Free

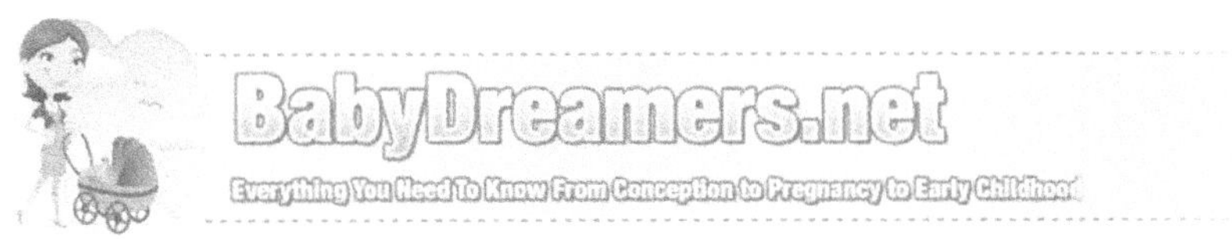

A Short Read is a type of book that is designed to be read in one quick sitting.

These no fluff books are perfect for people who want an overview about a subject in a short period of time.

Table of Contents

Is Your Lifestyle Affecting Your Fertility?

Is Your Lifestyle Affecting Your Fertility?

When it comes to fertility and reproductive health, the choices we make in our daily lives can have a significant impact. From our age to our habits, various factors can influence our ability to conceive and have a healthy pregnancy. In this article, we will explore the impact of lifestyle choices on fertility and reproductive health, shedding light on the importance of making informed decisions.

Age is one of the most crucial factors to consider when it comes to fertility. As women age, their egg quantity and quality decrease, making it more challenging to conceive. Similarly, men experience a decline in sperm count and motility as they get older. Therefore, it is essential to understand the correlation between age and fertility and the potential challenges it may present.

Another lifestyle choice that can have a detrimental effect on fertility is smoking. Both female and male smokers face specific risks and complications when trying to conceive. For women, smoking can disrupt hormonal balance, affect ovulation, and increase the risk of miscarriage. In men, smoking can lead to decreased sperm count and quality, reducing the chances of successful fertilization.

Alcohol consumption is another lifestyle factor that can impact fertility. Excessive alcohol intake can disrupt hormonal balance in women, affecting ovulation and increasing the risk of infertility. In men, alcohol can reduce sperm production and impair reproductive function. It is crucial to understand the relationship between alcohol and fertility and make informed choices.

Stress is a common part of modern life, but it can also take a toll on fertility. Psychological stress can contribute to infertility by disrupting hormonal balance and interfering with the reproductive process. Physical stressors, such as excessive exercise or significant weight fluctuations, can also affect fertility. Managing stress and finding healthy coping mechanisms are essential for optimizing chances of conception.

Diet plays a significant role in fertility, as a balanced and nutritious eating plan can support reproductive health. Women trying to conceive should ensure they are getting key nutrients, such as folic acid, iron, and omega-3 fatty acids, which are vital for reproductive function. Men's fertility can also be influenced by their diet, with nutrients like zinc and vitamin C playing a crucial role in sperm quality and quantity.

Environmental factors, such as exposure to harmful chemicals and endocrine-disrupting substances, can also impact fertility. Pesticides, industrial pollutants, and certain household products may interfere with reproductive function and increase the risk of infertility. Understanding the potential risks and taking necessary precautions is essential for protecting fertility.

Weight is another lifestyle factor that can affect fertility. Both obesity and being underweight can pose challenges when trying to conceive. Obesity increases the risk of conditions such as polycystic ovary syndrome (PCOS) and can disrupt hormonal balance. Being underweight can lead to irregular menstrual cycles and difficulties in achieving pregnancy. Maintaining a healthy body weight is crucial for optimizing fertility.

Exercise is beneficial for overall health, but intense exercise can have a negative impact on fertility. Intense physical activity can disrupt hormonal balance and menstrual cycles in women, making it more challenging to conceive. On the other hand, regular moderate exercise has been shown to have a positive effect on fertility and reproductive health. Finding the right balance is key.

Adequate sleep is essential for overall well-being, including reproductive function. Sleep deprivation can disrupt hormonal balance in both men and women, affecting fertility. Establishing healthy sleep habits and prioritizing sufficient rest can help optimize reproductive function.

Sexual health, including the risk of sexually transmitted infections (STIs), can also impact fertility. Certain STIs can lead to complications such as pelvic inflammatory disease (PID) or damage to the reproductive organs, increasing the risk of infertility. Practicing safe sex and regular STI screenings are essential for preserving fertility.

Lastly, certain medications can have an impact on fertility. Medications such as antidepressants, antihistamines, and painkillers may interfere with reproductive function. It is crucial to consult with a healthcare provider when planning for pregnancy to understand the potential effects of medications and make informed decisions.

In conclusion, our lifestyle choices can have a significant impact on fertility and reproductive health. Understanding the potential risks and making informed decisions is essential for optimizing chances of conception and having a healthy pregnancy. By taking care of our bodies and making conscious choices, we can support our fertility journey.

Age and Fertility

Age plays a significant role in fertility for both men and women. As individuals age, their reproductive capabilities naturally decline. For women, this decline is primarily due to a decrease in the number and quality of eggs. Women are born with a finite number of eggs, and as they age, the quantity and quality of these eggs diminish. This can make it more challenging to conceive and increases the risk of pregnancy complications.

For men, age also impacts fertility, although to a lesser extent than women. While men continue to produce sperm throughout their lives, the quality of their sperm may decrease with age. Older men may experience a decline in sperm count and motility, which can affect their ability to fertilize an egg. Additionally, advanced paternal age has been linked to an increased risk of certain genetic conditions in offspring.

It is important for individuals and couples to be aware of the impact of age on fertility when planning to start a family. Understanding the correlation between age and fertility can help individuals make informed decisions and seek appropriate medical assistance if needed. It is advisable to consult with a healthcare provider or fertility specialist to assess fertility potential and explore options for conception, such as assisted reproductive technologies.

Smoking and Fertility

Smoking and Fertility

Smoking has long been recognized as a major health hazard, but its detrimental effects extend beyond just respiratory problems and cancer. Research has shown that smoking can significantly impact fertility and reduce the chances of conception for both men and women.

For women, smoking can disrupt the delicate hormonal balance necessary for ovulation and implantation. It can also damage the reproductive organs, leading to issues such as blocked fallopian tubes and decreased egg quality. Women who smoke are more likely to experience difficulties in getting pregnant and have a higher risk of miscarriage.

In men, smoking can have a negative impact on sperm production and quality. It can lead to decreased sperm count, motility, and morphology, making it more difficult for sperm to reach and fertilize an egg. Smoking can also damage the DNA in sperm, increasing the risk of genetic abnormalities in offspring.

Furthermore, secondhand smoke can also affect fertility. Studies have shown that exposure to secondhand smoke can reduce fertility in both men and women, highlighting the importance of creating a smoke-free environment for those trying to conceive.

To increase the chances of conception and promote overall reproductive health, it is crucial for individuals and couples to quit smoking. Quitting smoking not only improves fertility but also enhances overall health and well-being. It is never too late to quit, and there are various resources and support available to help individuals kick the habit.

By eliminating smoking from your lifestyle, you can significantly improve your fertility and increase the likelihood of a successful pregnancy. Take control of your reproductive health and say goodbye to smoking for a brighter and healthier future.

Female Smokers and Fertility

Female smokers face numerous risks and complications when it comes to fertility and trying to conceive. Smoking has been linked to a variety of reproductive health issues in women, making it important to understand the potential consequences.

One of the main risks associated with smoking is a decrease in fertility. Studies have shown that smoking can disrupt the delicate hormonal balance in the female reproductive system, leading to irregular menstrual cycles and ovulation problems. This can make it more difficult for women to conceive naturally.

In addition to decreased fertility, smoking also increases the risk of pregnancy complications. Women who smoke are more likely to experience ectopic pregnancies, where the fertilized egg implants outside of the uterus. This can be a life-threatening condition and may result in the loss of the pregnancy.

Furthermore, smoking during pregnancy can have serious consequences for both the mother and the baby. It increases the risk of miscarriage, premature birth, low birth weight, and developmental issues in the baby. Secondhand smoke exposure can also be harmful, so it is important for women to avoid smoking environments even if they do not smoke themselves.

Quitting smoking is crucial for women who are trying to conceive or are already pregnant. It can improve fertility, reduce the risk of pregnancy complications, and promote a healthier environment for the developing baby. If you are a female smoker and planning to have a baby, consider seeking support and resources to help you quit smoking and improve your chances of a successful pregnancy.

Male Smokers and Fertility

Smoking is not only harmful to female fertility but also has a significant impact on male fertility. Research has shown that smoking can lead to decreased sperm count and quality, making it more difficult for men to conceive.

One of the main ways smoking affects male fertility is by reducing sperm production. The toxic chemicals in cigarettes can damage the DNA in sperm cells, leading to abnormalities and decreased motility. This can make it harder for sperm to reach and fertilize an egg, decreasing the chances of conception.

In addition to reduced sperm count and quality, smoking can also affect male reproductive hormones. Nicotine and other chemicals in cigarettes can disrupt hormone production, including testosterone. This can further impact fertility by affecting sperm development and function.

It is important for men who are trying to conceive to quit smoking or avoid exposure to secondhand smoke. Quitting smoking can help improve sperm count and quality, increasing the chances of successful conception. It is also advisable for men to adopt a healthy lifestyle, including regular exercise and a balanced diet, to further support reproductive health.

Alcohol and Fertility

Alcohol and fertility are closely linked, and it is important to understand the potential risks involved. While moderate alcohol consumption may not have a significant impact on fertility, excessive drinking can have detrimental effects on both men and women trying to conceive.

For women, alcohol can disrupt hormonal balance and affect ovulation. It can also increase the risk of miscarriage and decrease the chances of successful implantation. Heavy drinking during pregnancy can lead to fetal alcohol syndrome, which can cause developmental issues in the baby.

For men, alcohol can reduce sperm production and impair sperm quality. It can also lead to erectile dysfunction and hormonal imbalances that can affect fertility. Heavy drinking can decrease the chances of successful conception and increase the risk of genetic abnormalities in offspring.

It is important for couples trying to conceive to be aware of their alcohol consumption and consider making lifestyle changes if necessary. Limiting alcohol intake or avoiding it altogether can significantly improve fertility outcomes. It is also advisable to seek professional guidance and support if alcohol consumption is a concern.

Effects of Alcohol on Female Fertility

Alcohol consumption can have a significant impact on female fertility. When women consume alcohol, it can disrupt the delicate hormonal balance in their bodies, leading to irregular menstrual cycles and affecting ovulation. The liver plays a crucial role in metabolizing hormones, and excessive alcohol consumption can impair liver function, leading to hormonal imbalances that can interfere with the reproductive system.

Alcohol can also affect the quality and quantity of eggs produced by the ovaries. Studies have shown that alcohol consumption can decrease the number of eggs available for fertilization and increase the risk of chromosomal abnormalities in the eggs. This can make it more difficult for women to conceive and increase the chances of miscarriage if pregnancy does occur.

Furthermore, alcohol can interfere with the implantation of a fertilized egg in the uterus. It can affect the lining of the uterus, making it less receptive to implantation and increasing the risk of early pregnancy loss. Additionally, alcohol consumption during pregnancy can have severe consequences for the developing fetus, leading to fetal alcohol spectrum disorders and other birth defects.

It is important for women who are trying to conceive to be mindful of their alcohol consumption. It is recommended to limit or avoid alcohol altogether when trying to get pregnant. If you are struggling with alcohol addiction, seeking professional help and support is crucial for your overall health and fertility.

Effects of Alcohol on Male Fertility

The effects of alcohol on male fertility can be significant, with one of the key impacts being reduced sperm production. Alcohol consumption can disrupt the delicate hormonal balance in the body, leading to decreased sperm count and impaired sperm quality. This can make it more difficult for couples to conceive and increase the time it takes to achieve pregnancy.

Alcohol can also affect the structure and function of the male reproductive organs. Chronic alcohol use has been linked to testicular atrophy, which is the shrinkage of the testicles. This can further contribute to fertility issues by reducing the production of healthy sperm.

In addition to the direct effects on sperm production, alcohol can also impact sexual function. Excessive alcohol consumption can lead to erectile dysfunction and decreased libido, making it harder for men to engage in sexual activity and potentially reducing the chances of conception.

It is important for men who are trying to conceive to be mindful of their alcohol consumption. Limiting or avoiding alcohol altogether can help to improve male fertility and increase the chances of successful conception. It is advisable for men to discuss their alcohol use and any concerns about fertility with a healthcare provider, who can provide personalized guidance and support.

Stress and Fertility

Stress can have a significant impact on fertility and reproductive health. When we experience high levels of stress, our bodies release stress hormones such as cortisol, which can disrupt the delicate hormonal balance necessary for ovulation and conception. In women, stress can also affect the regularity and length of menstrual cycles, making it more difficult to predict fertile days.

Fortunately, there are strategies that can help manage stress and improve chances of conception. One effective approach is to incorporate stress-reducing activities into your daily routine. This can include practices such as yoga, meditation, deep breathing exercises, or even engaging in hobbies that bring you joy and relaxation. Taking time for self-care and prioritizing your mental and emotional well-being can have a positive impact on your fertility journey.

It's also important to seek support from your partner, friends, or a professional counselor if needed. Talking about your feelings and concerns can help alleviate stress and provide a sense of comfort and understanding. Additionally, maintaining a healthy lifestyle with regular exercise, a balanced diet, and adequate sleep can contribute to overall stress reduction and improve fertility.

Remember, everyone's fertility journey is unique, and it's essential to be patient and kind to yourself throughout the process. By managing stress effectively and adopting healthy coping mechanisms, you can optimize your chances of conception and create a nurturing environment for a healthy pregnancy.

Psychological Stress and Fertility

Psychological stress can have a significant impact on fertility. When individuals experience high levels of stress, it can disrupt the delicate hormonal balance necessary for reproductive function. Stress can affect both men and women, and it is important to understand the psychological factors that can contribute to infertility.

One of the main psychological factors that can affect fertility is anxiety. Constant worrying and feelings of anxiety can activate the body's stress response, leading to the release of stress hormones such as cortisol. Elevated levels of cortisol can interfere with the production of reproductive hormones, affecting ovulation in women and sperm production in men.

Another psychological factor that can contribute to infertility is depression. Research has shown that individuals who are depressed may have lower fertility rates compared to those who are not. Depression can disrupt the normal functioning of the reproductive system and decrease sexual desire, making it more difficult to conceive.

Coping with stress is crucial for individuals who are trying to conceive. There are various strategies that can help manage psychological stress and improve fertility. One effective method is practicing relaxation techniques such as deep breathing, meditation, or yoga. These techniques can help calm the mind and reduce stress levels.

Seeking support from loved ones or joining a support group can also be beneficial. Talking about one's feelings and concerns with others who are going through similar experiences can provide emotional support and alleviate stress. Additionally, engaging in activities that bring joy and relaxation, such as hobbies or spending time in nature, can help reduce stress levels.

It is important to remember that infertility is a complex issue, and psychological stress is just one factor that can contribute to difficulties in conceiving. If stress levels remain high or if there are other underlying medical conditions, it is recommended to seek professional help from a healthcare provider or a fertility specialist.

Physical Stress and Fertility

Physical stressors, such as excessive exercise or weight fluctuations, can have a significant impact on fertility. When the body is subjected to intense physical stress, it can disrupt the delicate balance of hormones and affect reproductive function.

Excessive exercise, especially when combined with inadequate nutrition, can lead to irregular menstrual cycles or even the absence of menstruation altogether. This is known as exercise-induced amenorrhea, and it can make it more difficult for women to conceive. The body may perceive the high levels of physical activity as a threat to survival, leading to a decrease in reproductive hormones.

On the other hand, rapid weight fluctuations, whether it's gaining or losing a significant amount of weight in a short period, can also impact fertility. Both obesity and being underweight can disrupt hormonal balance and interfere with ovulation. Women who are overweight may experience irregular menstrual cycles or have difficulty producing mature eggs, while those who are underweight may have irregular or absent periods.

It's important to find a balance when it comes to physical activity and maintaining a healthy weight. Moderate exercise can actually have a positive impact on fertility by improving blood circulation and reducing stress levels. However, it's crucial to avoid excessive exercise or extreme weight fluctuations, as they can negatively affect reproductive health.

If you're trying to conceive and suspect that physical stressors may be impacting your fertility, it's advisable to consult with a healthcare professional. They can provide guidance on finding the right balance of exercise and maintaining a healthy weight to optimize your chances of conceiving.

Diet and Fertility

Diet plays a crucial role in fertility, and maintaining a balanced and nutritious eating plan is essential for optimizing reproductive health. The food we consume provides the necessary nutrients for our bodies to function properly, including the reproductive system. A well-rounded diet can help regulate hormones, support healthy ovulation, and improve overall fertility.

When it comes to fertility, both men and women should focus on consuming a variety of nutrient-rich foods. For women, certain key nutrients are particularly important. These include folic acid, iron, calcium, and omega-3 fatty acids. Folic acid is essential for the development of a healthy baby and can be found in foods such as leafy greens, citrus fruits, and fortified cereals. Iron is important for blood production and can be found in foods like lean meats, beans, and spinach. Calcium is crucial for bone health and can be obtained from dairy products, leafy greens, and fortified plant-based milk alternatives. Omega-3 fatty acids, found in fatty fish, flaxseeds, and chia seeds, have been shown to support reproductive health.

For men, certain nutrients are also vital for maintaining optimal reproductive health. These include zinc, selenium, vitamin C, and vitamin E. Zinc is involved in sperm production and can be found in foods like oysters, beef, and pumpkin seeds. Selenium is an antioxidant that helps protect sperm from damage and can be obtained from foods like Brazil nuts, tuna, and eggs. Vitamin C is essential for sperm motility and can be found in citrus fruits, strawberries, and bell peppers. Vitamin E is another antioxidant that supports sperm health and can be found in foods like almonds, sunflower seeds, and spinach.

In addition to these specific nutrients, it is important to follow a balanced and nutritious eating plan overall. This means including a variety of fruits, vegetables, whole grains, lean proteins, and healthy fats in your diet. Avoiding processed foods, excessive sugar, and unhealthy fats is also recommended for optimal fertility.

It is worth noting that achieving a healthy weight through diet is also important for fertility. Both being underweight and overweight can have negative effects on reproductive health. Maintaining a healthy body weight through a balanced diet and regular exercise can help regulate hormones and improve fertility.

In summary, diet plays a significant role in fertility. A balanced and nutritious eating plan that includes key nutrients for both men and women is essential for optimizing reproductive health. By focusing on consuming a variety of nutrient-rich foods and maintaining a healthy weight, individuals can support their fertility and increase their chances of conception.

Key Nutrients for Female Fertility

When it comes to female fertility, certain key nutrients play a crucial role in optimizing reproductive health and increasing the chances of conception. These essential nutrients not only support the overall functioning of the reproductive system but also contribute to hormonal balance and the development of a healthy pregnancy.

One of the most important nutrients for female fertility is folate, also known as folic acid. Folate is essential for the production of DNA and RNA, which are vital for the development of a healthy fetus. It is particularly important during the early stages of pregnancy to prevent neural tube defects. Good sources of folate include leafy green vegetables, citrus fruits, beans, and fortified cereals.

Another key nutrient for female fertility is iron. Iron is necessary for the production of hemoglobin, which carries oxygen to the reproductive organs and supports the development of healthy eggs. Iron deficiency can lead to anemia, which can negatively impact fertility. Good sources of iron include lean meats, poultry, fish, beans, and fortified grains.

Omega-3 fatty acids are also essential for female fertility. These healthy fats help regulate hormone production, reduce inflammation, and promote optimal egg development. Good sources of omega-3 fatty acids include fatty fish like salmon and sardines, flaxseeds, chia seeds, and walnuts.

Vitamin D is another important nutrient for female fertility. It plays a role in regulating menstrual cycles and promoting ovulation. Additionally, vitamin D deficiency has been linked to infertility and pregnancy complications. Sun exposure is the best source of vitamin D, but it can also be found in fatty fish, fortified dairy products, and egg yolks.

Lastly, antioxidants such as vitamin C and vitamin E are crucial for female fertility. These nutrients help protect the reproductive cells from oxidative stress and DNA damage, improving the quality of eggs and supporting a healthy pregnancy. Good sources of antioxidants include fruits and vegetables, especially berries, citrus fruits, and leafy greens.

It's important to note that while these nutrients can support female fertility, they should not be considered a cure-all for underlying fertility issues. It's always recommended to consult with a healthcare provider or fertility specialist for personalized advice and guidance.

Key Nutrients for Male Fertility

When it comes to male fertility, certain nutrients play a crucial role in maintaining reproductive health and optimizing sperm quality and quantity. These key nutrients provide the necessary building blocks for sperm production and function, as well as support overall reproductive function.

1. Zinc: Zinc is an essential mineral that is vital for male fertility. It plays a critical role in sperm development and maturation, as well as in maintaining healthy testosterone levels. Good food sources of zinc include oysters, beef, poultry, pumpkin seeds, and spinach.

2. Selenium: Selenium is another important nutrient for male fertility. It is a powerful antioxidant that helps protect sperm from oxidative damage and supports healthy sperm motility. Good dietary sources of selenium include Brazil nuts, tuna, sardines, and eggs.

3. Vitamin C: Vitamin C is a potent antioxidant that helps protect sperm from oxidative stress and improves sperm quality. It also plays a role in enhancing sperm motility. Citrus fruits, strawberries, kiwi, and bell peppers are excellent sources of vitamin C.

4. Vitamin E: Vitamin E is another antioxidant that helps protect sperm cells from damage. It also plays a role in maintaining healthy sperm membrane integrity. Good sources of vitamin E include almonds, sunflower seeds, spinach, and avocados.

5. Omega-3 fatty acids: Omega-3 fatty acids, particularly docosahexaenoic acid (DHA), are essential for sperm health. They support sperm membrane integrity, enhance sperm motility, and promote overall reproductive function.

Fatty fish like salmon, sardines, and mackerel are rich sources of omega-3 fatty acids.

6. Coenzyme Q10: Coenzyme Q10 is a powerful antioxidant that helps protect sperm cells from oxidative damage. It also supports energy production in sperm cells, which is crucial for their motility and function. Good dietary sources of coenzyme Q10 include organ meats, fish, and soybean oil.

7. L-arginine: L-arginine is an amino acid that plays a role in sperm production and quality. It is involved in the synthesis of nitric oxide, which helps relax and dilate blood vessels, improving blood flow to the reproductive organs. Good food sources of L-arginine include meat, poultry, dairy products, and nuts.

8. Vitamin D: Vitamin D deficiency has been associated with decreased sperm quality and fertility issues. Adequate vitamin D levels are essential for optimal reproductive function in men. Sun exposure and fortified foods like milk and cereals are good sources of vitamin D.

9. B vitamins: B vitamins, particularly folate (B9), B12, and B6, are important for male fertility. They help support DNA synthesis and integrity in sperm cells. Good dietary sources of B vitamins include whole grains, legumes, leafy greens, and lean meats.

10. Antioxidants: In addition to specific nutrients, a diet rich in antioxidants can help protect sperm cells from oxidative damage and improve overall sperm health.

Antioxidant-rich foods include berries, dark chocolate, green tea, and colorful fruits and vegetables.

It's important to note that while these nutrients can support male fertility, they are not a guarantee of conception. A balanced and varied diet, along with a healthy lifestyle, is key to optimizing reproductive health. If you're concerned about your fertility or are planning to conceive, it's always a good idea to consult with a healthcare provider or a fertility specialist for personalized advice and guidance.

Environmental Factors and Fertility

Environmental factors play a significant role in fertility, as exposure to toxins and pollutants can have detrimental effects on reproductive health. The modern world is filled with various chemicals and pollutants that can disrupt the delicate balance of our hormonal systems and interfere with the natural processes of conception and pregnancy.

Chemical exposure is a major concern when it comes to fertility. Pesticides used in agriculture, industrial pollutants, and even everyday household products can contain harmful chemicals that have been linked to reproductive issues. These chemicals can accumulate in the body over time and affect both men and women.

Endocrine-disrupting chemicals (EDCs) are of particular concern in relation to fertility. These substances can mimic or interfere with the hormones in our bodies, leading to hormonal imbalances and reproductive problems. EDCs can be found in plastic products, personal care items, and even in the air we breathe.

To reduce the impact of environmental factors on fertility, it is important to minimize exposure to harmful chemicals. This can be achieved by opting for organic and natural products, avoiding the use of pesticides and insecticides, and being mindful of the air quality in your environment. Additionally, maintaining a healthy lifestyle and supporting your body's natural detoxification processes can help reduce the accumulation of toxins in the body.

By being aware of the potential impact of environmental toxins and pollutants on fertility, individuals and couples can take proactive steps to protect their reproductive health and increase their chances of conception.

Chemical Exposure and Fertility

Chemical exposure can have a significant impact on fertility, with harmful chemicals like pesticides and industrial pollutants posing potential risks. These substances can interfere with reproductive processes and disrupt hormonal balance, leading to difficulties in conceiving.

Pesticides, commonly used in agriculture to control pests and weeds, have been linked to fertility issues in both men and women. Studies have shown that exposure to pesticides can affect sperm quality and motility in men, while in women, it can disrupt hormonal regulation and interfere with ovulation. Additionally, certain pesticides have been associated with an increased risk of miscarriage and birth defects.

Industrial pollutants, such as heavy metals and chemicals found in air and water pollution, can also have adverse effects on fertility. These substances can accumulate in the body over time and impair reproductive function. For example, exposure to lead, mercury, or cadmium has been linked to decreased sperm quality and increased risk of infertility in men. In women, exposure to pollutants like polychlorinated biphenyls (PCBs) and dioxins can disrupt the menstrual cycle and interfere with the implantation of a fertilized egg.

It is important to be aware of potential sources of chemical exposure and take necessary precautions to minimize risks. This may include using protective equipment when working with chemicals, avoiding or limiting exposure to pesticides and industrial pollutants, and ensuring proper ventilation in work and living environments. Regular monitoring and testing for chemical exposure can also be beneficial in assessing potential risks to fertility.

When planning for pregnancy, it is advisable to consult with a healthcare provider or fertility specialist to understand the potential impact of chemical exposure on fertility and discuss strategies to minimize risks. They can provide guidance on lifestyle modifications, such as dietary changes and detoxification protocols, to support reproductive health and increase the chances of successful conception.

Endocrine Disruptors and Fertility

Endocrine disruptors are chemicals that can interfere with the normal functioning of the endocrine system, which plays a crucial role in regulating fertility and reproductive health. These chemicals mimic or block the actions of natural hormones in the body, leading to hormonal imbalances and potential fertility issues.

There are various sources of endocrine disruptors that individuals may come into contact with on a daily basis. Some common sources include:

- Pesticides and herbicides used in agriculture
- Industrial pollutants, such as dioxins and polychlorinated biphenyls (PCBs)
- Plasticizers, such as bisphenol A (BPA) found in certain plastics
- Phthalates used in personal care products and plastics
- Certain medications, such as hormone replacement therapy drugs

These endocrine-disrupting chemicals can enter the body through various routes, including ingestion, inhalation, and skin contact. Once inside the body, they can accumulate and disrupt the normal hormonal balance, potentially leading to fertility problems.

Research has shown that exposure to endocrine disruptors can have adverse effects on both male and female fertility. In women, these chemicals can interfere with ovulation, disrupt the menstrual cycle, and affect the quality of eggs.

In men, they can reduce sperm count, impair sperm motility, and affect sperm quality.

It is important to be aware of the potential sources of endocrine disruptors and take steps to minimize exposure. This can include choosing organic produce, using natural and chemical-free personal care products, avoiding plastic containers that contain BPA, and reducing exposure to environmental pollutants.

Consulting with a healthcare provider can also be helpful in understanding the potential risks and taking appropriate measures to protect fertility. They can provide guidance on lifestyle changes, recommend fertility-friendly products, and offer advice on minimizing exposure to endocrine disruptors.

Weight and Fertility

Weight plays a significant role in fertility, and maintaining a healthy body weight is crucial for both men and women who are trying to conceive. Being either overweight or underweight can have detrimental effects on reproductive health and decrease the chances of successful pregnancy.

Obesity, defined as having a body mass index (BMI) of 30 or higher, can pose various challenges when it comes to fertility. It can disrupt hormonal balance, leading to irregular menstrual cycles and ovulation problems in women. Additionally, obesity is associated with an increased risk of conditions such as polycystic ovary syndrome (PCOS), which can further impact fertility. In men, obesity can lead to a decrease in sperm quality and quantity, making it more difficult to achieve pregnancy.

On the other hand, being underweight, typically characterized by a BMI below 18.5, can also affect fertility. Women who are underweight may experience irregular or absent menstrual cycles, as well as difficulties in ovulation. In men, being underweight can lead to a decrease in sperm production and quality, reducing the chances of successful conception.

It is important to note that weight-related fertility issues are not solely limited to women. Men's weight can also have an impact on reproductive health and fertility. Maintaining a healthy weight through a balanced diet and regular exercise is essential for both partners when trying to conceive.

To optimize fertility, it is recommended to consult with a healthcare provider or fertility specialist who can provide personalized guidance based on individual circumstances. They can help assess body weight and provide recommendations for achieving and maintaining a healthy weight. In some cases, medical interventions or lifestyle modifications may be necessary to address weight-related fertility issues.

In conclusion, weight plays a significant role in fertility, and maintaining a healthy body weight is crucial for both men and women. Whether it is obesity or being underweight, imbalances in weight can impact reproductive health and decrease the chances of successful pregnancy. Seeking professional guidance and adopting a healthy lifestyle can help optimize fertility and increase the likelihood of conception.

Obesity and Fertility

Obesity can have a significant impact on fertility and the ability to conceive. When trying to get pregnant, individuals who are obese may face various challenges and increased risks. Obesity is defined as having a body mass index (BMI) of 30 or higher, and it can affect both men and women.

For women, obesity can disrupt hormonal balance and interfere with the regularity of menstrual cycles. This can make it more difficult to predict ovulation and time intercourse effectively. Additionally, obesity is associated with an increased risk of conditions such as polycystic ovary syndrome (PCOS) and insulin resistance, which can further complicate fertility.

Obesity in men can also impact fertility. It can lead to hormonal imbalances, such as reduced testosterone levels, which can affect sperm production and quality. Studies have shown that obese men may have lower sperm counts and decreased sperm motility, making it more challenging to achieve pregnancy.

Furthermore, obesity is linked to an increased risk of pregnancy complications, such as gestational diabetes, preeclampsia, and cesarean delivery. These risks not only affect the health of the mother but can also impact the well-being of the baby.

It's important for individuals who are obese and trying to conceive to take steps to manage their weight and improve their overall health. This may involve adopting a balanced and nutritious diet, engaging in regular physical activity, and seeking guidance from healthcare professionals. By addressing obesity and making positive lifestyle changes, individuals can improve their chances of successful conception and have a healthier pregnancy.

Underweight and Fertility

Being underweight can have a significant impact on fertility and can pose potential difficulties when trying to achieve pregnancy. When a person's body weight falls below the healthy range, it can disrupt hormonal balance and affect reproductive function.

One of the key factors affected by being underweight is the menstrual cycle. Irregular or absent periods are common in women who are underweight, which can make it challenging to track ovulation and determine the most fertile days for conception. Additionally, underweight women may have lower levels of estrogen, a hormone essential for healthy ovulation and the development of the uterine lining.

Furthermore, being underweight can lead to a decrease in the production of certain hormones necessary for fertility, such as luteinizing hormone (LH) and follicle-stimulating hormone (FSH). These hormones play crucial roles in the maturation and release of eggs from the ovaries.

In men, being underweight can also have adverse effects on fertility. Low body weight can lead to a decrease in testosterone levels, which is essential for sperm production. This can result in a reduced sperm count and poor sperm quality, making it more challenging to achieve pregnancy.

It is important for individuals who are underweight and trying to conceive to focus on gaining a healthy amount of weight through a balanced and nutritious diet. This includes consuming adequate amounts of protein, healthy fats, and carbohydrates to support reproductive function. Consulting with a healthcare provider or a registered dietitian can be beneficial in developing a personalized meal plan and ensuring proper nutrient intake.

In addition to addressing weight concerns, it is crucial to address any underlying medical conditions that may be contributing to being underweight. Conditions such as eating disorders, thyroid dysfunction, or malabsorption issues should be evaluated and treated by a healthcare professional to optimize fertility.

Overall, being underweight can have significant effects on fertility and can make it more challenging to achieve pregnancy. It is essential to maintain a healthy body weight through proper nutrition and address any underlying medical conditions to improve the chances of conception.

Exercise and Fertility

Exercise plays a crucial role in maintaining overall health and well-being, and it also has a significant impact on fertility and reproductive health. Finding the optimal balance between exercise and fertility is essential for individuals who are trying to conceive.

Regular physical activity has been shown to improve fertility outcomes in both men and women. For women, exercise can help regulate hormonal balance, promote healthy ovulation, and enhance the chances of conception. It can also improve blood flow to the reproductive organs, ensuring optimal conditions for fertilization and implantation.

However, it is important to note that intense exercise or excessive physical exertion can have a negative impact on fertility. High levels of exercise can disrupt the delicate hormonal balance in the body, leading to irregular menstrual cycles and decreased fertility. It is crucial to find a balance and avoid overexertion, especially for women who are actively trying to conceive.

On the other hand, moderate exercise has been found to have numerous benefits for fertility. Engaging in regular, moderate-intensity exercise can help reduce stress levels, improve overall cardiovascular health, and enhance fertility outcomes. It is recommended to aim for at least 150 minutes of moderate-intensity exercise per week, such as brisk walking, swimming, or cycling.

It is important to listen to your body and make adjustments to your exercise routine as needed. If you are experiencing difficulties conceiving or have any concerns about the impact of exercise on your fertility, it is advisable to consult with a healthcare professional who specializes in reproductive health. They can provide personalized guidance and recommendations based on your specific circumstances.

Intense Exercise and Fertility

Intense exercise can have a significant impact on fertility and menstrual cycles. While regular moderate exercise is beneficial for reproductive health, engaging in intense physical activity can potentially disrupt the delicate balance of hormones necessary for fertility.

Excessive exercise can lead to irregular or absent menstrual cycles, a condition known as exercise-induced amenorrhea. This occurs due to the suppression of the reproductive hormones estrogen and progesterone, which are essential for ovulation and the preparation of the uterus for pregnancy. Without a regular menstrual cycle, it becomes more challenging to conceive.

In addition to irregular periods, intense exercise can also contribute to other fertility-related issues. Women who engage in excessive physical activity may experience a decrease in the production of cervical mucus, which plays a crucial role in supporting sperm survival and transportation. This can make it more difficult for sperm to reach and fertilize the egg.

Moreover, intense exercise can lead to hormonal imbalances, such as elevated levels of stress hormones like cortisol. These hormonal disruptions can interfere with the regular release of eggs from the ovaries and affect the overall quality of the eggs produced. As a result, the chances of successful fertilization and implantation may be reduced.

It is important for women who are trying to conceive to find a balance between exercise and fertility. While staying active and maintaining a healthy weight is beneficial, it is essential to avoid excessive or intense exercise routines that may negatively impact reproductive health. Consulting with a healthcare provider or fertility specialist can provide guidance on appropriate exercise levels and help optimize fertility.

Benefits of Moderate Exercise for Fertility

Regular moderate exercise has been shown to have numerous benefits for fertility and overall reproductive health. Engaging in moderate physical activity on a regular basis can help regulate hormone levels, improve blood circulation to the reproductive organs, and reduce stress levels, all of which can contribute to increased fertility.

One of the key benefits of moderate exercise for fertility is its ability to help maintain a healthy body weight. Obesity and being underweight can both have negative effects on fertility, so finding the right balance is important. Moderate exercise can help individuals achieve and maintain a healthy weight, which in turn can improve fertility outcomes.

In addition to weight management, moderate exercise can also improve ovulation in women. Regular physical activity has been shown to enhance the regularity of menstrual cycles and promote healthy ovulation. This can increase the chances of conception and improve overall reproductive health.

Furthermore, moderate exercise can help reduce stress levels, which can have a significant impact on fertility. High levels of stress can disrupt hormonal balance and interfere with the reproductive system. Engaging in regular exercise releases endorphins, which are natural mood boosters, and can help alleviate stress and promote a positive mindset.

It is important to note that moderation is key when it comes to exercise and fertility. Intense and excessive exercise can actually have a negative impact on fertility by disrupting hormonal balance and causing irregular menstrual cycles. It is recommended to engage in moderate exercise for about 30 minutes to an hour most days of the week.

Examples of moderate exercises that can benefit fertility include brisk walking, swimming, cycling, and yoga. These activities are low-impact and can be easily incorporated into daily routines. It is always advisable to consult with a healthcare provider before starting any new exercise regimen, especially for individuals with pre-existing medical conditions or fertility concerns.

In conclusion, regular moderate exercise can have a positive impact on fertility and overall reproductive health. It can help maintain a healthy weight, improve ovulation, reduce stress levels, and promote a positive mindset. By incorporating moderate exercise into your daily routine, you can increase your chances of conception and improve your overall reproductive well-being.

Sleep and Fertility

Sleep plays a crucial role in maintaining overall health and well-being, and it also has a significant impact on fertility. Adequate sleep is essential for reproductive function and can affect both men and women's ability to conceive. When we sleep, our bodies undergo various restorative processes that are necessary for optimal reproductive health.

One of the key ways sleep influences fertility is through hormonal regulation. Sleep deprivation or inadequate sleep can disrupt the delicate balance of hormones involved in the reproductive system. For women, irregular sleep patterns or insufficient sleep can affect the production of hormones necessary for ovulation and menstrual regularity. In men, lack of sleep can lead to decreased sperm production and quality.

Additionally, sleep deprivation can contribute to increased stress levels, which can further impact fertility. Chronic stress can disrupt the hormonal signals necessary for successful conception and can even lead to irregular menstrual cycles in women. It's important to establish healthy sleep habits to optimize fertility and reproductive function.

Effects of Sleep Deprivation on Fertility

Sleep deprivation can have a significant impact on fertility in both men and women. When we don't get enough sleep, it can disrupt the delicate hormonal balance in our bodies, which is essential for reproductive function. Hormones such as estrogen, progesterone, and testosterone play a crucial role in regulating the menstrual cycle, sperm production, and ovulation. For women, sleep deprivation can lead to irregular menstrual cycles and ovulation problems. It can also affect the quality of eggs released during ovulation, making it more difficult to conceive. In men, lack of sleep can result in decreased testosterone levels and reduced sperm quality and quantity. This can impair fertility and decrease the chances of successful conception. Additionally, sleep deprivation can contribute to chronic stress, which further affects fertility. Stress hormones, such as cortisol, can interfere with the production of reproductive hormones and disrupt the normal functioning of the reproductive system. To optimize fertility, it is important to prioritize sleep and establish healthy sleep habits. Aim for 7-9 hours of uninterrupted sleep each night and create a relaxing bedtime routine. Avoid electronic devices before bed, as the blue light emitted can interfere with sleep patterns. Create a comfortable sleep environment, keep the room dark and quiet, and maintain a consistent sleep schedule. If you are experiencing difficulties conceiving, it is important to consult with a healthcare provider who can provide guidance and support. They can help identify any underlying sleep disorders or hormonal imbalances that may be impacting fertility and recommend appropriate treatments or lifestyle changes. Remember, getting enough sleep is not only important for overall health and well-being but also plays a crucial role in optimizing fertility. Take the time to prioritize sleep and create a sleep-friendly environment to support your reproductive health.

Establishing Healthy Sleep Habits for Fertility

Establishing Healthy Sleep Habits for Fertility

Getting enough quality sleep is crucial for optimizing fertility and reproductive health. Sleep plays a vital role in regulating hormones, including those involved in the menstrual cycle and sperm production. If you're trying to conceive, it's important to prioritize healthy sleep habits to maximize your chances of success.

Here are some strategies to improve sleep quality and duration:

- **Stick to a consistent sleep schedule:** Try to go to bed and wake up at the same time every day, even on weekends. This helps regulate your body's internal clock and promotes better sleep.
- **Create a relaxing bedtime routine:** Establish a soothing routine before bed to signal to your body that it's time to wind down. This can include activities such as reading a book, taking a warm bath, or practicing relaxation techniques like deep breathing.
- **Create a sleep-friendly environment:** Make your bedroom a sanctuary for sleep by keeping it cool, dark, and quiet. Consider using blackout

curtains, earplugs, or a white noise machine to block out any disruptions that may interfere with your sleep.

- **Avoid electronic devices before bed:** The blue light emitted by smartphones, tablets, and computers can interfere with your body's natural sleep-wake cycle. Try to limit your exposure to electronic devices at least an hour before bedtime.

- **Limit caffeine and alcohol intake:** Both caffeine and alcohol can disrupt sleep patterns and negatively impact fertility. It's best to avoid or limit consumption of these substances, especially in the hours leading up to bedtime.

- **Manage stress:** High levels of stress can make it difficult to fall asleep and stay asleep. Incorporate stress-reducing activities into your daily routine, such as yoga, meditation, or journaling, to promote relaxation and better sleep.

- **Exercise regularly:** Engaging in regular physical activity can improve sleep quality and duration. However, it's important to avoid intense exercise close to bedtime, as it may energize your body and make it harder to fall asleep.

By implementing these strategies, you can establish healthy sleep habits that support optimal fertility. Remember, quality sleep is an essential component of overall reproductive health, so prioritize it as part of your journey to conceive.

Sexual Health and Fertility

Sexual health plays a crucial role in fertility and reproductive health. The connection between sexual health, sexually transmitted infections (STIs), and fertility is an important aspect to consider for individuals trying to conceive. STIs can have a significant impact on reproductive health and can lead to complications that affect fertility.

When it comes to fertility, certain STIs can cause damage to the reproductive organs, such as the fallopian tubes and the uterus in women, and the testicles and the vas deferens in men. This damage can result in infertility or increase the risk of ectopic pregnancies, where the fertilized egg implants outside the uterus. Additionally, untreated STIs can lead to pelvic inflammatory disease (PID), which can cause scarring and blockages in the reproductive organs.

Preventive measures are crucial for maintaining sexual health and preserving fertility. Safe sex practices, such as using condoms and practicing monogamy, can help reduce the risk of contracting STIs. Regular screenings for STIs are also important, as early detection and treatment can prevent complications and minimize the impact on fertility.

If you suspect you may have an STI or are planning to conceive, it is important to consult with a healthcare provider. They can provide guidance on appropriate testing, treatment options, and steps to take to optimize fertility. Open and honest communication with your partner and healthcare provider is key to ensuring sexual health and fertility are prioritized.

Impact of STIs on Fertility

Sexually transmitted infections (STIs) can have a significant impact on fertility and reproductive health. These infections are transmitted through sexual contact and can affect both men and women. It is important to be aware of the potential complications and risks associated with STIs in order to protect your fertility.

One of the main concerns with STIs is their ability to cause inflammation and damage to the reproductive organs. In women, certain STIs like chlamydia and gonorrhea can lead to pelvic inflammatory disease (PID), which can cause scarring and blockages in the fallopian tubes. This can make it difficult for the egg to travel from the ovaries to the uterus, increasing the risk of infertility or ectopic pregnancy.

In men, STIs can also cause inflammation and damage to the reproductive system. For example, untreated gonorrhea can lead to epididymitis, which is the inflammation of the epididymis, a tube that carries sperm. This can result in reduced sperm count and motility, affecting the chances of conception.

Furthermore, certain STIs, such as human papillomavirus (HPV) and herpes, can cause genital warts and ulcers. These can lead to discomfort and pain during sexual intercourse, making it more challenging for couples to conceive naturally.

It is important to note that not all STIs have visible symptoms, which is why regular screenings and practicing safe sex are crucial. Early detection and treatment of STIs can help minimize the risk of complications and protect your fertility.

In conclusion, the impact of STIs on fertility should not be taken lightly. It is important to prioritize sexual health, practice safe sex, and seek medical attention if you suspect you may have an STI. By doing so, you can protect your reproductive health and increase your chances of conceiving when the time is right.

Preventive Measures for Sexual Health and Fertility

Preventive Measures for Sexual Health and Fertility

When it comes to maintaining sexual health and preserving fertility, taking preventive measures is essential. By practicing safe sex and undergoing regular screenings for sexually transmitted infections (STIs), individuals can protect their reproductive health and increase their chances of conceiving.

Safe Sex Practices

Engaging in safe sex practices is crucial for preventing the transmission of STIs and protecting fertility. This includes using barrier methods of contraception, such as condoms, which provide a physical barrier against STIs. It is important to use condoms consistently and correctly to reduce the risk of infection.

Additionally, limiting sexual partners and ensuring that both partners have been tested for STIs before engaging in sexual activity can further reduce the risk of transmission. Open and honest communication with sexual partners about sexual health is also essential for maintaining a healthy and safe sexual relationship.

Regular STI Screenings

Regular screenings for STIs are vital for early detection and treatment, which can prevent long-term complications and protect fertility. It is recommended that sexually active individuals, especially those planning to conceive, undergo regular screenings for common STIs such as chlamydia, gonorrhea, syphilis, and HIV.

These screenings can be done at healthcare clinics, sexual health centers, or through private healthcare providers. Early detection of STIs allows for prompt treatment, reducing the risk of complications that can negatively impact reproductive health.

Conclusion

By prioritizing safe sex practices and regular STI screenings, individuals can take proactive steps towards

preserving their sexual health and fertility. These preventive
measures not only protect against the transmission of STIs
but also contribute to overall reproductive well-being.
Remember, open communication, responsible sexual
behavior, and regular screenings are key to maintaining
optimal sexual health and increasing the chances of
achieving a healthy pregnancy.

Medications and Fertility

When it comes to fertility, it's important to consider the
potential effects of certain medications. Medications can
have various impacts on fertility, both positive and negative.
Understanding these effects and considering them when
trying to conceive is crucial for individuals and couples.

Some medications can directly affect reproductive health
and fertility. For example, certain medications used to treat
chronic conditions like autoimmune disorders or cancer may
have fertility-related side effects. These medications can
interfere with hormonal balance, disrupt menstrual cycles,
or affect sperm production. It's essential to consult with a
healthcare provider to understand the potential impact of
these medications on fertility and explore alternative options
if necessary.

Additionally, other medications that are commonly used for
different purposes, such as antidepressants, antihistamines,
or painkillers, may also have indirect effects on fertility.
While the impact of these medications on fertility may vary,
it's important to discuss their use with a healthcare provider
when planning for pregnancy. They can provide guidance

on potential risks and offer alternatives that are safer for
fertility.

Common Medications and Fertility

Common Medications and Fertility

When it comes to fertility, certain medications can have an
impact on both men and women. It's important to be aware
of the potential effects of medications such as
antidepressants, antihistamines, and painkillers, as they can
potentially interfere with reproductive health.

Antidepressants, commonly prescribed for mental health
conditions such as depression and anxiety, have been
associated with changes in hormone levels and sexual
function. While the exact impact on fertility is still being
studied, it's important to discuss any concerns with your
healthcare provider if you are planning to conceive.

Antihistamines, often used to manage allergies and cold
symptoms, may cause drying of cervical mucus, making it
more difficult for sperm to reach the egg. This can
potentially affect fertility, especially for couples trying to
conceive. It's advisable to consult with your doctor about
alternative options or strategies if you are regularly using
antihistamines and planning for pregnancy.

Painkillers, including nonsteroidal anti-inflammatory drugs
(NSAIDs) and opioids, are commonly used to manage pain.
While occasional use is generally considered safe,
prolonged or excessive use of these medications may have

an impact on fertility. NSAIDs have been shown to interfere with ovulation and implantation, while opioids can disrupt hormone production and affect sperm quality. If you are regularly using painkillers and trying to conceive, it's important to discuss this with your healthcare provider to explore alternative pain management options.

It's important to remember that every individual is unique, and the impact of medications on fertility can vary. If you have concerns about the medications you are taking and their potential effects on your fertility, it's always best to consult with your healthcare provider. They can provide personalized advice and guidance based on your specific situation.

Consulting with a Healthcare Provider

When planning for pregnancy, it is crucial to consult with a healthcare provider regarding medication use. Medications can have varying effects on fertility and the development of a healthy pregnancy. It is essential to have open and honest discussions with your healthcare provider to ensure that you are making informed decisions.

During these consultations, it is important to provide your healthcare provider with a comprehensive list of all the medications you are currently taking, including prescription drugs, over-the-counter medications, and any supplements or herbal remedies. This information will help your healthcare provider assess the potential risks or benefits associated with these medications and make recommendations tailored to your specific situation.

It is worth noting that some medications can have adverse effects on fertility or increase the risk of birth defects. For example, certain antidepressants, antihistamines, and painkillers have been associated with decreased fertility or potential harm to the developing fetus. By discussing these medications with your healthcare provider, you can explore alternative options or adjust your treatment plan to minimize any potential risks.

Your healthcare provider can also provide guidance on the timing of medication use in relation to conception. In some cases, it may be necessary to discontinue certain medications before attempting to conceive, while in other situations, it may be safe to continue taking them. Your healthcare provider will consider the specific medication, your medical history, and your individual circumstances to provide personalized recommendations.

Remember, the goal is to optimize your chances of conceiving and maintaining a healthy pregnancy. Your healthcare provider is an invaluable resource who can provide expert advice and support throughout your journey to parenthood. By consulting with them and discussing your medication use, you can make informed decisions that prioritize both your fertility and the well-being of your future child.

Frequently Asked Questions

- **Q: How does age affect fertility?**

Get How To Be A Super Mom - 100% FREE

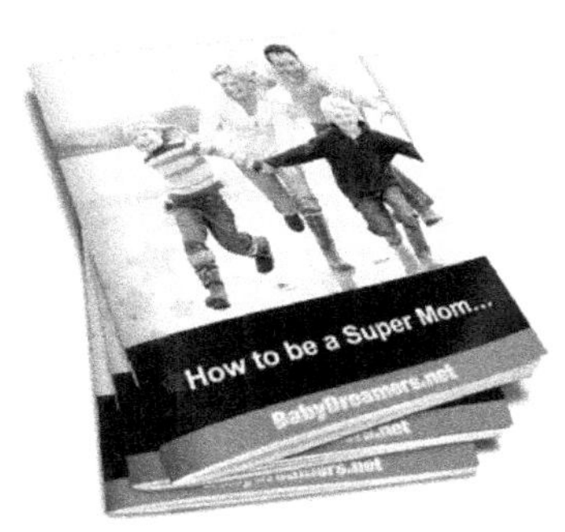

For being one of our amazing readers, we would love to offer you another book we have created, 100% free.

Being a mom is probably the most important job in the world – we've all heard that, and it's true. You're bringing up the next generation of wonderful, intelligent, loving, creative, responsible people.

We all want to be Super Mom and to be everything and do everything, but it this possible?

Being a Super Mom is possible, but you have to learn how to empower yourself to be the kind of Super Mom that you feel you need to be, keeping in mind that the title Super Mom doesn't mean the same thing to everyone.

Get How to be a Super Mom For Free at

BabyDreamers.net